BLACK MEDICINE:
The Dark Art of Death

BLACK MEDICINE:
The Dark Art of Death
by
N. Mashiro, Ph.D.

*The Vital Points of the Human Body
In Close Combat*

Library of Congress Cataloging in Publication Data
Mashiro, N.
  Black Medicine.
  Includes bibliographical references.
  1. Hand-to-hand fighting. 2. Hand-to-hand fighting,
Oriental. 3. Self-defense. I. Title.
GV1111.M358   613.6'6   78-2210
ISBN 0-87364-101-9

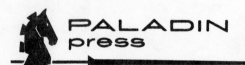

PALADIN
press

Post Office Box 1307
Boulder, Colorado 80306

TABLE OF CONTENTS

FOREWORD

The title **Black Medicine** is a word play on "black magic." Just as white magic does good, and black magic specializes in evil, there is a white medicine which cures and a black kind of medical and anatomical knowledge that is used to produce injuries and death. Black medicine is the study of the "vital points" of human anatomy for the purpose of disrupting the structure and physiology of the body in the most rapid and deadly manner possible.

This manual is devoted to the discussion of one hundred and seventy parts of the human body where a minimum amount of force will produce a maximum impact on a person's ability to fight. The study of these vital points is basic to all branches of the martial arts. This particular discussion is oriented toward the karate or self-defense student, the police officer, and the military combat specialist to whom a thorough grounding in the details of human anatomy may make a life-or-death difference someday.

There are several reasons for studying the vital points of the body. Self-defense students, because they expect to use their skills only against high odds (or not at all), need every advantage they can get. Karateists, with their highly developed power and accuracy, can obtain amazing results by utilizing the vital points as targets and therefore have a responsibility to be familiar with these weak points of the body if only to avoid injuring their friends during practice sessions. Law officers have a serious responsibility to study the vital points carefully because such knowledge makes a small amount of force go a long way, minimizing cries of "police brutality" and increasing an officer's chances of survival in the street. Members of the armed forces, remembering some of the lessons of Viet Nam, study the vital areas as a kind of close-quarters insurance. After all, the M-16 doesn't always fire when you want it to . . . .

There will be some people who will suggest that the macabre material in this manual should not be made public because of the use to which is might be put by criminals. My reply is that *they already know* . . . from cruel and gruesome experience. It is the rest of us who are morally restrained from acquiring first-hand knowledge who need instructions. To those of you who read this manual with a sense of shock, horror, and rising nausea I dedicate this book. Someday it may save one of your lives.

N. Mashiro
May 1978

Introduction

Power of blows: A few words of introduction are in order, particularly for those readers who are not very familiar with the martial arts. Although many of the vital points listed in this manual would obviously be effective when attacked by anyone, there are others which only a highly trained martial artist can use. The reader will note that occasionally a vital point is designated for "an extremely powerful blow." This refers to the punch, chop or kick of a black belt who can break three one-inch boards with a punch, or crack a brick with the side of his hand. The author has occasionally amused his friends by neatly slicing coconuts in two with the "knife edge" of his hand, and he has no doubts about what would happen if he applied the same blow to the side of someone's head. If you do not have the ability to deliver such attacks you should either restrict yourself to the targets which require less power or learn to use hand-held weapons.

Speed of blows: A second factor which seems almost incredible to those not involved in the martial arts is the speed with which blows can be delivered by a trained fighter. Even a mediocre karateist can stand with his hands at his sides and without warning deliver an incapacitating punch to his opponent's groin in 1/25 of a second. Flurries of punches to the face and body can be generated at upwards of six punches per second. There are even a few gifted individuals who can get off six *kicks* in one second!

Hand-held weapons: The weapons referred to at various places within the text are the pistol, hatchet, machete, bowie knife, stilletto, bayonet, ice pick, nightstick and yawara stick. Most of these are self-explanatory. The bayonet is presumed to be fixed on the end of a rifle. The yawara stick, for the uninitiated, is a short rod about the size of a ballpoint pen which is clenched in the fist with both ends protruding.

General comments: Basically, the goal of attacking the vital points is to make the opponent *stop what he is doing*. You attack his vital points to force him to *stop* trying to injure you — *stop* choking you — *stop* holding you — *stop* raping you —

or *stop* hurting someone else. There are three general ways to accomplish this:

(1) Make him lose his concentration. If he stops thinking about hitting you he will stop trying to hit you.

(2) Interfere with his control over his body. If he has a bruised nerve in his arm and cannot form a fist, he can't hit you.

(3) Destroy the integrity of his body. If his forearm is broken, he won't try to hit you whether he can form a fist or not!

If the thing the enemy must stop doing is "stop living," which will be the case for some readers, there are again three ways to accomplish the end:

(1) Destroy the central nervous system. Damage to the brain, brain stem, or spinal cord is usually fatal and always incapacitating.

(2) Destroy or interfere with circulation. Draining the circulatory system of blood is an indirect attack on the brain, as is closing off the carotid arteries. Injuring the heart is another approach.

(3) Interfere with breathing. Either strangulation or injury to the lungs, filling them with blood, is effective.

The reader should be aware that the terms "fatal" and "lethal" have a special meaning in some military manuals. In the military context a knock-out blow is "fatal" because it makes the enemy helpless under circumstances where the victor could not afford to show any mercy. Under such circumstances, the difference between being helpless and being dead is just a matter of seconds. In this manual these words are employed in their conventional meanings.

One of the most important lessons which a study of the vital areas reveals is that there are vulnerable targets almost everywhere on the body. If any part of your opponent is close enough to strike, you can hurt him, (Figure 1).

This discussion is oriented toward the adult male body. The targets are 99% similar in the female. The difference lies in that the breasts are much more sensitive to injury in the female, and of course a woman has no testicles. In addition, the bones of the female are smaller and lighter than those of the male, and are easier to break.

Figure 1

The diagrams were prepared under the assumption that the reader would not need any help finding his eyeball, nose, lip, fingers, testicles, etc. Therefore, most of the illustrations concentrate on the vital points which are harder to locate. In the event that both the text and the illustrations fail to convey a clear description of the location of the target, the reader is advised to consult a standard medical anatomy text such as Gray's Anatomy.

Figure 1 is a general diagram of all the vital points covered by this manual. By carefully reading the description in each paragraph of the text, you should have no difficulty locating the appropriate point on the diagram. Figure 1 has been left without identifying labels partly for clarity, and partly so that copies of the diagram may be used as examination sheets in self-defense and karate classes.

Notice that although the concentration of vital points in the head and neck is very high, the overall distribution is fairly even throughout the body. It is important to know this, because it means that if *any* part of the opponent is within reach, *you can hurt him.*

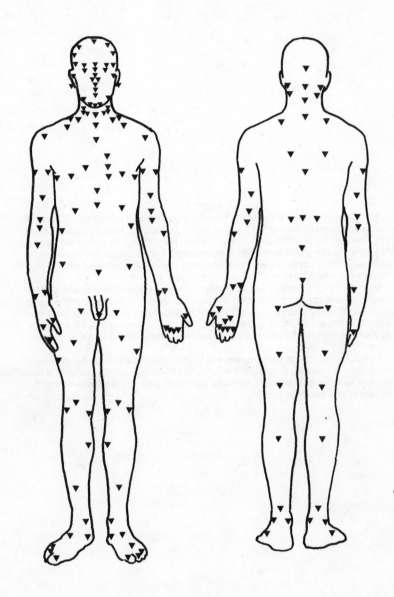

FIGURE 1

12

Vital Points of the Head

Hair: There are several releases and throws which depend on tearing or pulling at an opponent's hair. The pain can be used as a distraction, or a grip on the hair may be used to control the motion of the head. An example would be to grasp the opponent's hair with both hands and pull his head down sharply into your rising knee.

Bregma: The point near the top of the skull where the frontal and parietal bones meet. A violent, hammer-like blow from a fist dislocates the frontal bone, causing severe damage to the motor areas of the brain which lie immediately beneath. There is a ranger trick involving hitting a sentry over the head with his own helmet which uses this striking point, (Figure 2).

Coronal suture: The posterior edge of the frontal bone, passing from the temples diagonally up to the bregma; the joint between the frontal bone and each parietal bone. Strictly speaking this includes the bregma, and the mechanism of injury is much the same, except that the lateral aspects of the coronal suture are vulnerable to a blow from the side such as a karate chop or a blow from a nightstick, (Figure 2).

Temporal bone: The side of the skull above and around the ear is fairly thick and not a very good target. Most people have an instinctive tendency to strike this region, however, if they are called on to use a club or nightstick. There is some evidence that this is an innate behavior pattern over a million years old, and self-defense students have to learn to overcome the impulse. There are much better places to apply a nightstick if necessary. On the other hand, a hatchet can make quite an impression on the temporal bone, (Figure 2).

Sphenoid bone: The sphenoid bone is a small patch of bone on the side of the head about an inch back from the eye. A relatively thin bone, it is the only bone of the brain case which is concave inward, making it structurally weak. A potentially lethal target, the sphenoid bone can be attacked by a variety of blows, and is very vulnerable to a yawara stick or ice pick, (Figures 2 and 3).

Temporal artery: A knife slash to the side of the head over the sphenoid bone can sever the temporal artery. This is a

Figure 2

Figure 2 is a diagram of the head, throat, and part of the upper shoulder. The location of the letters on the drawing represents the location of the point to strike. The reader should realize that many structures have been left out of this diagram for purposes of clarity, particularly in the region of the throat.

a. Bregma
b. Coronal suture
c. Temporal bone (the large bone above it is the parietal bone)
d. Sphenoid bone
e. Orbital bones (the entire area around the eye)
f. Glabella
g. Nasal bones
h. Nose
i. Philtrum (or intermaxillary suture)
j. Mouth (just below the lower gum line)
k. Mandible
l. Point of chin
m. Occipital bone
n. Vertebral artery (note rings of bone)
o. Carotid sinus (in the carotid artery. Note the position of this point relative to the angle of the jaw and the level of the thyroid cartilage. The vagus nerve and the jugular vein run parallel to this artery, between it and the skin.)
p. Thyroid cartilage
q. Trachea
r. 3rd intervertebral space
s. Brachial plexus
t. Subclavian artery (behind collar bone)

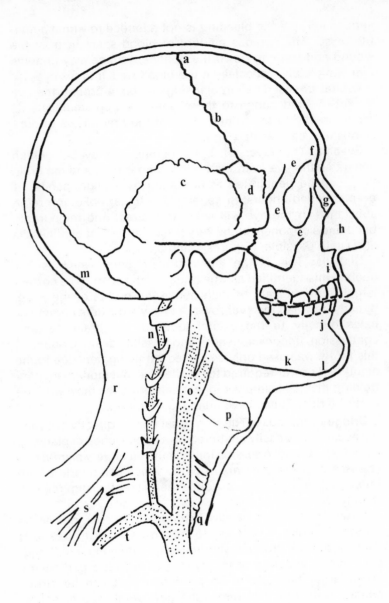

FIGURE 2

serious injury if the bleeding is not attended to within a minute or so. The copious amount of blood spurting from the wound and running down the opponent's face may unnerve him completely, especially if the blood runs into his eyes.

Orbital bones: The circular ridge of bone around the eye socket. A solid punch to these bones will communicate its force directly to the frontal lobes of the brain. Loss of consciousness can result, (Figure 2).

Eyeball: The layer of bone behind the eyeball which separates the eye from the brain is paper-thin, and the brain case can be penetrated at this point by a knife, pencil, or even stiffened fingers. In general, any finger poke or foreign substance in the eye will serve to distract and temporarily blind one's opponent at the very least. Permanent blindness is also quite possible, (Figures 4 and 5).

Glabella: This is the lethal striking point which is frequently mis-identified as "the bridge of the nose." The correct target is about half an inch above the bridge of the nose, directly between the eyebrows. A heavy blow here communicates directly to the frontal lobes of the brain, causing concussion, unconsciousness and possibly death. Originally, this target was used only by skilled karate fighters due to the amount of power required to be effective, but modern military training manuals simply suggest delivering the blow with the butt of a rifle. Times have changed, (Figure 2).

Bridge of the nose: The thin nasal bones, directly between the eyes, can be easily shattered by a punch, chop or glancing club blow. It is not a serious injury, but can be very painful and releases copious amounts of blood which can interfere with breathing. It can also produce permanent disfigurement, (Figure 2).

Nose: The nose is heavily loaded with nerves, due to its sensory function. A light slap to the nose will cause no serious damage but will produce stunning pain, and temporary blindness due to watering of the eyes. The nose is a particularly good target because of its prominence. It can be struck equally well from five directions (left, right, above, below, straight in), and its position in the center of the face makes it a good target for a blow delivered with the back of the head against an opponent who is trying to pin one's arms from behind, (Figure 2).

Nostrils: Jamming your finger up to the second knuckle into

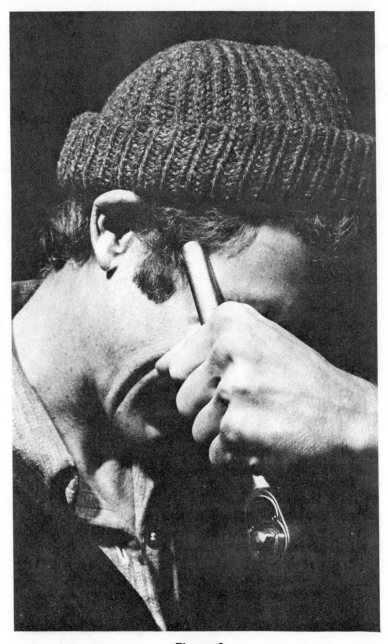

Figure 3
The yawara stick strike to the sphenoid bone (temple). Almost any small rod-shaped object can be used as a yawara stick.

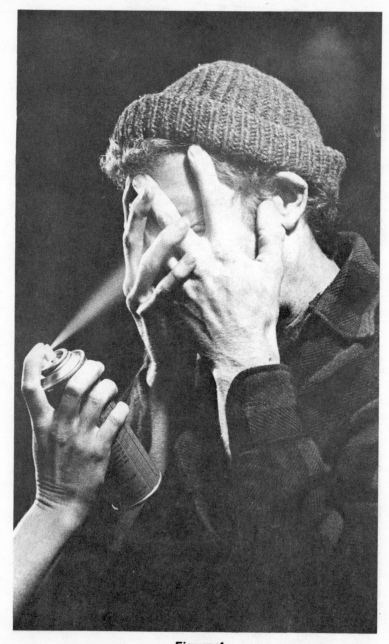

Figure 4
An extremely effective attack is to spray deodorant, insecticide, oven cleaner, hair spray or paint into an opponent's eyes, blinding him.

your opponent's nostril is a sure way to distract him and make him let go of you. For maximum effect bend your finger into a hook before yanking it back out! (Figures 2 and 5).

Philtrum or Intermaxillary suture: This is the upper lip just above the gum line, or about one quarter inch below the nose. A blow at this point commonly results in broken upper teeth, possibly some disruption of the nasal bones, and concussion to the brain since the upper jaw bones (maxilla) are firmly attached to the brain case. Less frequently a powerful karate punch to this point can generate shearing forces strong enough to fracture the *dens,* a small finger of bone which helps keeps the skull in place on top of the vertebral column. Trauma to the brain stem causes instant death, (Figure 2).

Lower lip: By twisting the lower lip between the thumb and index finger, twisting it through a half turn and pulling roughly you can make a drunk follow you anywhere. (Make *sure* he's drunk first!)

Mouth: Taken here to mean the point in the center of the mandible about one half inch below the lower lip (i.e., the gum line of the lower incisors). A blow here will cut the lip against the teeth or break off the lower teeth altogether, with the shock of impact being carried to the balancing organs in the inner ear through the mandible itself. Fossil evidence in vertebrate paleontology shows that the three tiny bones of the ear mechanism were once part of the mandible, hence the close relationship between the jaw and the ear. The shock to the ear disrupts balance and results in disorientation, dizziness, or unconsciousness, (Figure 2).

Mandible or Jaw: The lower edge of the jaw, about two inches from the point of the chin. Depending on the direction and force of the blow, the jaw may absorb the shock itself by dislocating or fracturing, or it may communicate the shock upwards through the teeth to the brain. The jaws lends itself to being attacked from below, as in the case of an uppercut, but its shape and size make it one of the most resistant bones in the body. A punch to the jaw always carries with it the possibility of injury to the attacker's fist, (Figures 2 and 6).

Point of chin: The point of the chin is vulnerable to a rising palm-heel attack or a rising elbow blow, either of which can be powerful enough to cause whiplash injury to the neck. It is also possible to dislocate the skull from the top of the spinal column, causing instant death, (Figure 2).

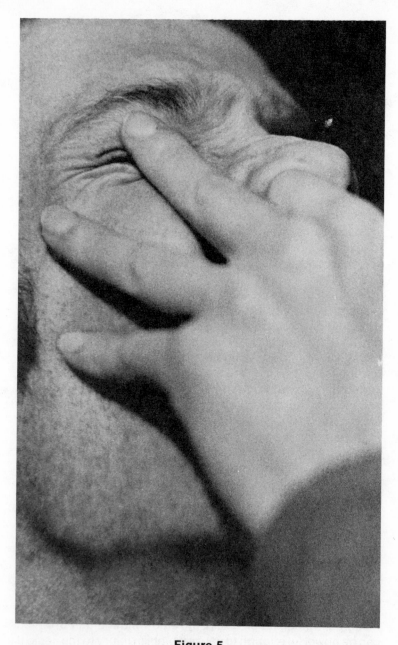

Figure 5
A finger jammed into a nostril is very painful. As the photo shows, this attack can easily be an attack on the eyes at the same time. A person subjected to this attack immediately tries to break away.

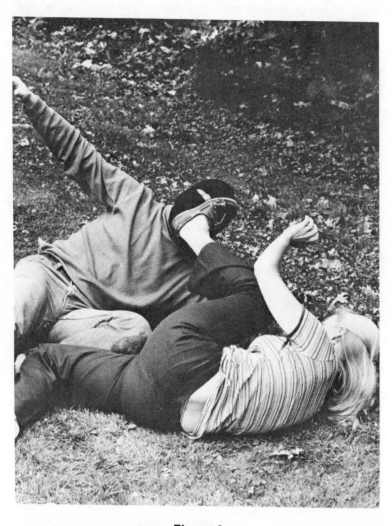

Figure 6
The heel-kick to the rapist's jaw illustrated here is an extremely powerful attack which involves no risk of injury to the woman. Had she tried to punch him in the face she might easily have broken her hand or wrist in the process.

Occipital bone (cerebellum): The attack point is in the center of the back of the head at the point where the trapezius muscles attach to the occipital bone (where you can feel the dome of the skull disappearing into the neck muscles). A blow to this area will cause concussion to the cerebellum, which is the portion of the brain concerned with the coordination of muscular movements and posture. This is a favorite target of assassins who specialize in hatchet work, (Figure 2).

Tympanum or Eardrum: The ear contains a high concentration of sensory nerves associated with hearing and balance. Striking the ear with a cupped hand sends a shock wave down the ear canal which ruptures the tympanum and shocks the delicate inner ear mechanisms, producing severe pain, dizziness, or unconsciousness. A pencil, ice pick or stilletto rammed into the ear has an even more dramatic effect.

Ear lobe: Under certain circumstances, the ear lobe can be seized in the teeth and even torn off, severely distracting the opponent. Women can use this technique to dissuade a drunk from amorous advances, (Figure 7).

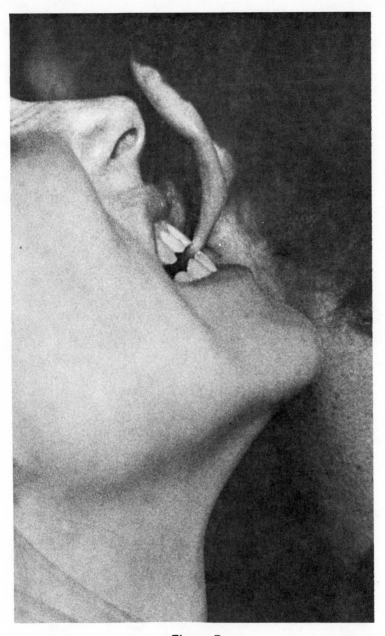

Figure 7
When a woman finds herself in an unwelcome embrace it is usually difficult for her to break free but very easy to get closer. Clamping on to the masher's ear with her teeth turns the tables . . . he then tries to push her away!

Vital Points of the
Neck and Throat

Facial nerve: The facial or seventh cranial nerve emerges from the skull just beneath the ear canal, from which position it branches out to supply the muscles of the face which control facial expressions. A knuckle blow to the soft spot immediately beneath the ear will bruise this nerve, producing startlingly severe pain and possibly some disorientation due to the shock to the inner ear. This point is frequently used as a "releaser," in that a coordinated attack on the left and right facial nerves will disconcert a masher or strangler sufficiently to allow his victim to escape. A gouge at this point with a yawara stick is very effective, (Figure 8).

Vertebral artery: There is a rare but always fatal injury which can accompany a blow to the side of the neck, especially if the blow lands just below the mastoid process of the skull, below and behind the ear. The vertebral artery, an important supplier of the brain, runs up the side of the neck through *rings of bone* attached to the cervical vertebrae. If struck in exactly the right way, this artery can be severed where it passes through a bone ring. The result is immediate unconsciousness followed by certain death. Surgical aid cannot come in time to prevent the death of the parts of the brain supplied by this artery, (Figure 2).

Hypoglossal nerve: This cranial nerve lies just inside the lower edge of the mandible slightly forward of the angle of the jaw. A sharp jab under the jaw at this point (as with stiffened fingers or yawara stick) will cause considerable pain.

Sternocleidomastoid muscle and the **Accessory nerve:** The accessory nerve is the eleventh cranial nerve, which innervates the sternocleidomastoid muscle and trapezius muscles. The first is the muscle which extends from the mastoid process behind the ear down to the clavicle and the sternum; the second is the muscle running between the top of the shoulder and the vertebrae of the neck which is used in shrugging the shoulders. A jab or gouge which catches the sternocleidomastoid about halfway down its length (about an inch below the angle of the jaw), will bruise both the muscle and accessory nerve, resulting in pain and partial temporary paralysis of

25

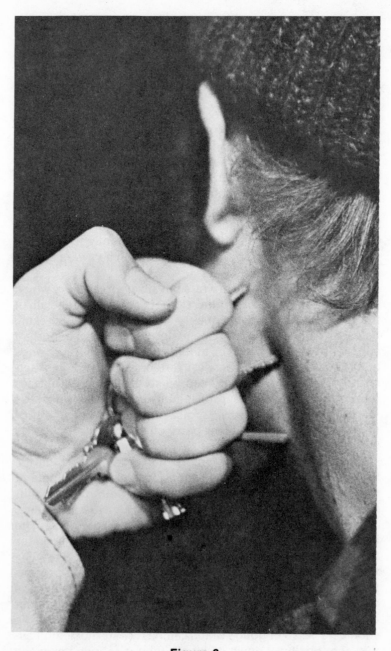

Figure 8
Car keys can be used to attack the facial nerve where it lies against the back of the jawbone.

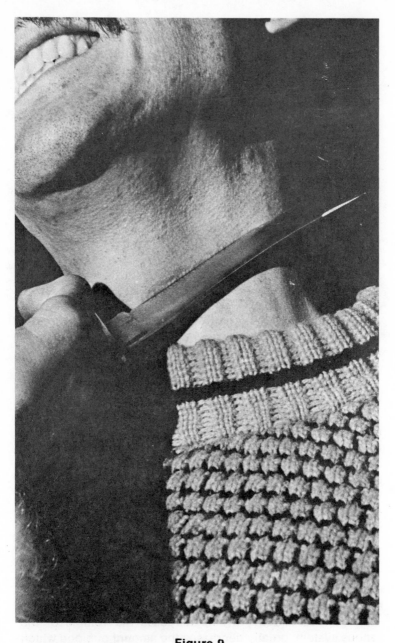

Figure 9
The jugular vein and the carotid artery are vulnerable to knife attack from about the position illustrated up to the level of the jaw. The slash should be about one and one-half inches deep to catch both vessels.

the neck and shoulders.

Jugular vein and the **Carotid artery:** A knife slash or saber cut across the side of the neck directly below the angle of the jaw will sever the jugular vein and, if deep enough, the carotid artery as well.

Fairbairn's timetable indicates unconsciousness within five seconds, and "death" in twelve seconds for this injury. This requires some qualification. Cutting off the blood supply to the brain for twelve seconds will not produce death or even brain injury, as every serious judo student knows. Brain deterioration requires one and one-half minutes or more of oxygen deprivation. Fairbairn's twelve second figure may indicate that after that period of time the victim has lost too much blood to be able to recover. If any first aid is to be applied it must come before this time limit, (Figures 9 and 10).

Carotid sinus and **Vagus nerve:** This is one of the most interesting of the karate striking points because of the sophistication of the effect which a light blow to this area can have. Since the brain is probably the most delicate organ in the body, and since it requires a constant and uniform flow of blood in order to function properly, the body has developed extraordinary safeguards to insure that the flow of blood to the brain is not interrupted. Similarly, the blood pressure to the brain must not be allowed to rise to too high a level because of the danger of cerebral hemorrhage. To maintain this *status quo* there have developed special nerve cells in the carotid artery called baroreceptors whose sole function is to monitor the blood pressure in this important artery. If the pressure suddenly rises to a high level, these baroreceptors respond by sending immediate signals to the central nervous system. Within a fraction of a second the central nervous system has acted in turn to decrease blood pressure in the body by causing four things to happen:

(1) The heart immediately slows down.

(2) With each beat the heart is able to pump out less blood.

(3) The artereolar smooth muscle relaxes, which greatly increases the volume of the arterial system, drawing blood away from the head.

(4) Venous dilation, which increases the volume of the venous system, greatly decreases the amount of blood which can get back to the heart.

The net result is an almost instantaneous four-way reaction

28

No.	Name of Artery	Size	Depth below Surface in inches	Loss of Consciousness in seconds	Death
1....	Brachial	Medium	½	14	1½ Min.
2....	Radial	Small	¼	30	2 "
3....	Carotid	Large	1½	5	12 Sec.
4....	Subclavian	Large	2½	2	3½ "
5....	(Heart)	—	3½	Instantaneous	3 "
6....	(Stomach)	--—	5	Depending on depth of cut	

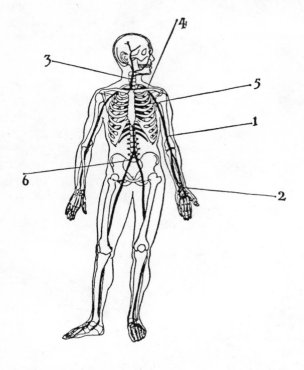

Figure 10

This is a reproduction of Captain W. E. Fairbairn's table of arterial targets for knife fighting as it appears in his combat manual, *Get Tough!* The source of Fairbairn's information is not clear, and the meaning of the times listed under the "Death" column apparently stand for the amount of time that can pass before the victim has lost too much blood to be able to recover. Death follows within minutes, much less rapidly than indicated in the table. The "Loss of Consciousness" figures seem quite reasonable, however.

29

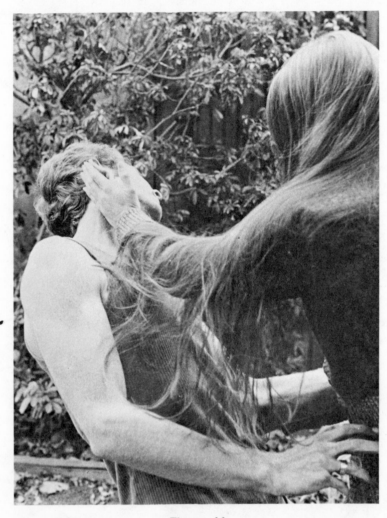

Figure 11
The blow to the bifurcation of the carotid artery is easy to apply and produces fainting, dizziness or disorientation without permanent injury.

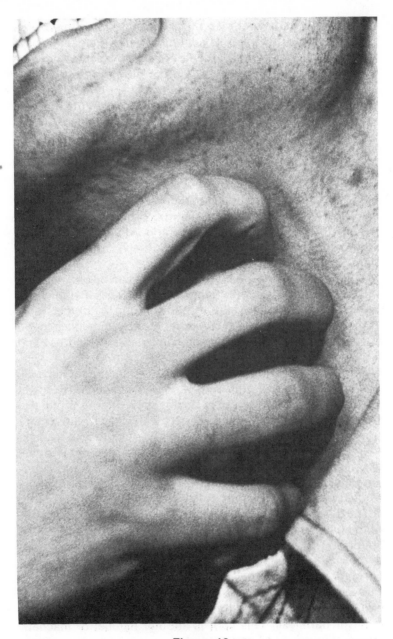

Figure 12
The thyroid cartilage can be crushed by a strong grip or by any of a variety of blows. Light pressure is extremely painful, and heavier pressure is extremely dangerous.

to decrease the flow of blood to the brain. This is the reason that the side of the neck is such an effective striking point, because shock to the baroreceptors forces the central nervous system to react (mistakenly) as if the blood pressure in the head had suddenly risen to a dangerously high level. The central nervous system responds with a drastic drop in blood pressure, and within a second or two the blood supply to the brain is cut off completely. Fainting is immediate and unavoidable, and yet the helpless victim has actually suffered no more than having a slightly bruised neck.

The vagus nerve, which runs beside the carotid artery at this point, is also involved in this reaction as it controls or affects the function of the pharynx, larynx, bronchi, lungs, heart, esophagus, stomach, intestines and kidneys. The blow momentarily disrupts control of all these organs at once, (Figures 2 and 11).

Thyroid cartilage: The thyroid cartilage can be crushed by a relatively light blow, after which the resulting hemorrhage swells the soft tissue of the throat until the windpipe swells shut and the victim dies of suffocation. Only immediate medical aid can prevent a horrible death in this case, (Figures 2 and 12).

Jugular notch: This is the "soft spot" in the front of the neck just above the manubrium. At this point the trachea is exposed to attack, being covered only by the skin, with no protective bones or muscles. A finger poke here will result in pain; a more powerful attack can crush the trachial cartilages and result in death by strangulation. A jab by a knife or bayonet into this spot spills blood into the trachea, which due to a reflex seizure makes it impossible for the victim to breathe. He chokes to death on his own blood, (Figures 2 and 13).

Third intervertebral space: The striking point is the center of the back of the neck where the column of vertebrae is least supported by surrounding tissues and is therefore weakest. A blow to this region produces severe trauma to the spinal cord, resulting in unconsciousness or death. TV heroes make free use of the chop to the back of the neck to knock out the bad guys, but in real life the technique is frequently fatal, and is never harmless. This spot is another hatchet or machete target, (Figures 2, 14 and 16).

Seven cervical vertebra: This is the last vertebra of the neck, resting immediately on top of the first thoracic vertebra. The

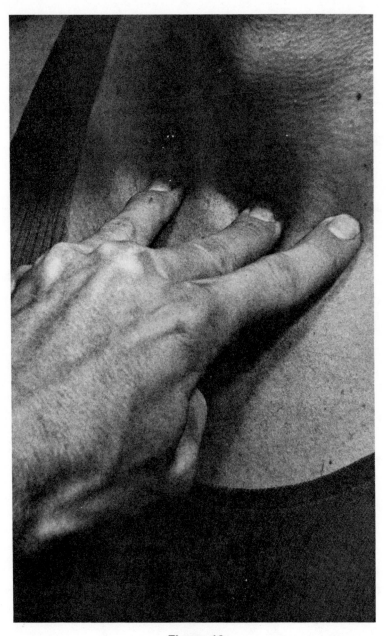

Figure 13
The three-finger strike to the throat. The tracheal cartilages lie just beneath the middle finger. (The index and ring fingers help locate the target in the dark.)

33

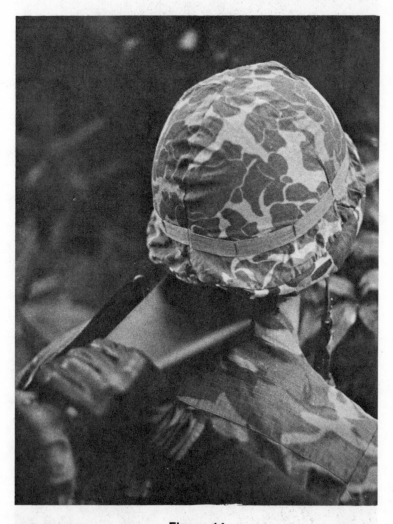

Figure 14
The blow to the third cervical vertebra administered to the back of a sentry's neck by the butt of a rifle.

first thoracic vertebra is braced into position by the first pair of ribs and by the muscles of the shoulder girdle, while the seventh cervical vertebra is not particularly braced in any way. For this reason the spinal cord may be attacked relatively easily at this point because the immobility of the first thoracic vertebra predisposes the system to a shearing injury between the two vertebrae. The seventh cervical vertebra also possesses an unusually long dorsal spine, which is vulnerable to painful fracture. This is the part of the neck under attack during a violent application of a Full Nelson hold, but is best attacked by a sharp, hammer-like blow of the fist, (Figure 16).

Figure 15

Figure 15 is a diagram of the vital points of the rib cage. The ribs are numbered downward from the top. White areas represent bone, while striated areas represent bands of elastic cartilage.

a. Manubrium
b. Sternal angle
c. Body of the sternum
d. Intercostal spaces (knife thrust to heart)
e. Xiphoid process
f. 5th and 6th ribs
g. 4th intercostal space
h. 7th intercostal space (costal cartilages)
i. Floating ribs
j. 1st lumbar vertebra

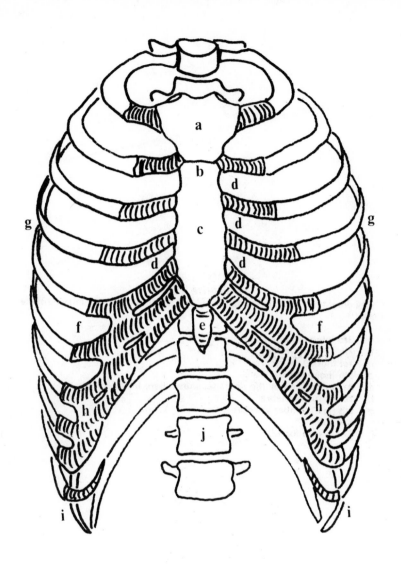

FIGURE 15

Figure 16

The diagram is of the entire spinal column as viewed from the left side of the body.

- a. 3rd intervertebral space
- b. 7th cervical vertebra
- c. 1st thoracic vertebra
- d. 5th thoracic vertebra
- e. Area occupied by the rib cage, shown here for reference
- f. 1st lumbar vertebra
- g. 5th (last) lumbar vertebra
- h. Sacrum
- i. Coccyx (tailbone)

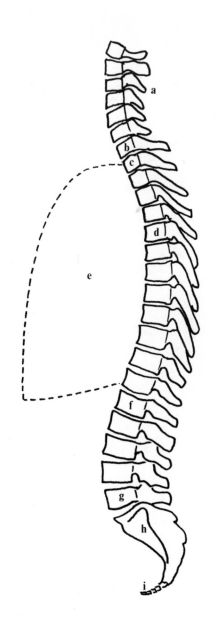

FIGURE 16

39

40

Vital Points of the Upper Trunk

Brachial plexus: This is beneath the muscle reaching from the top of the shoulder up to the vertebrae of the neck. A downward blow here can inhibit the muscles of the neck, shoulder and arm, severely limiting the opponent's ability to fight. In addition, a man can be forced to release a hold by pinching and gouging deep beneath this muscle with the thumb and fingers. Note: One should not expect the spectacular results obtained by *Star Trek's* Mr. Spock, (Figures 2 and 17).

Subclavian artery: A stilletto forced downward into the top of the shoulder in the soft spot behind the collarbone will sever the subclavian artery. The victim bleeds to death in seconds. This is a very difficult area to reach with a knife because it involves holding the weapon above the victim's shoulder and stabbing downward, an approach not widely endorsed by knife wielders, (Figure 2).

Clavicle or **Collar bone:** This is the prominent horizontal bone in the front of each shoulder. A heavy fist blow or sharp tap with a nightstack can snap it in two, effectively destroying the opponent's ability to fight with his hands, and in most cases completely putting him out of the fight. The jagged ends of the fracture may even be driven backward to penetrate the subclavian artery, which lies just behind the bone. Damage to this artery can be fatal, depending on the nature of the internal wounds.

Sternal angle: This is the point where the manubrium and the body of the sternum come together, about two inches below where the collar bones meet at the base of the throat. It is a weak point in the sternum, and if attacked with a powerful blow to the sternal "shield" over the heart, bronchus, lungs and thoracic nerves can be broken, producing pain and shock to the circulatory and respiratory systems. This crushing of the chest should produce unconsciousness at the very least and can be fatal. This injury is the reason automobiles are now supplied with collapsible steering columns to avoid chest damage in collisions, (Figure 15).

Intercostal spaces: There are four intercostal spaces next

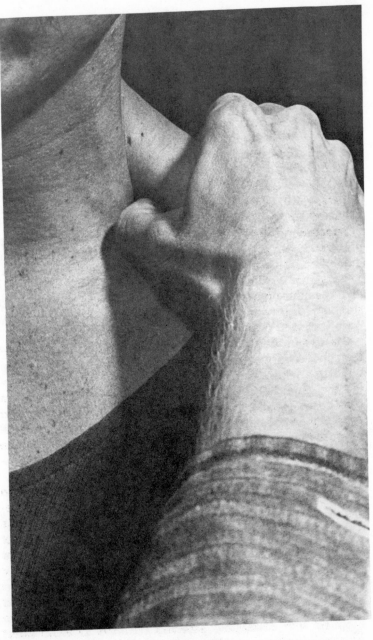

Figure 17
A very deep pinch into the trapezius muscle can bruise the bracial plexus, temporarily paralyzing the arms and shoulders. It is usually used as a release.

to the body of the sternum through which a stilletto point can be inserted into the heart. These are below the third, fourth and fifth rib on the left side, and below the fourth rib on the right. The blade should be angled in toward the midline of the body and jerked back and forth for maximum effect, (Figure 15).

Xiphoid process: A finger-like tab of cartilage hanging off the lowermost edge of the sternum. This is the insertion of the rectus abdominus muscle on the sternum. A powerful karate blow which strikes the xiphoid process while traveling upward at an angle toward the heart causes severe bruising to the liver, stomach and heart, resulting in unconsciousness or even death. This is also another knife route to the heart, (Figure 15).

Fifth and Sixth Ribs: The target area is about one inch below the nipple on either side. A powerful punch or a sharp kick at this point will breach the rib cage and inflict injuries on the lungs. This is the point where the fifth and sixth ribs articulate with the costal cartilages, the articulation being at the very tip of the bony part of the rib. Hence a blow at this point exerts maximum leverage against the ribs, fracturing them relatively easily, (Figure 15).

Sympathetic trunk: The striking point is the head of the third rib, right between the spine and the top of the shoulder blade. A powerful blow here will dislocate the rib, forcing it into the chest cavity. This tears the thick bundle of sympathetic nerves which lie next to the spine, and the rib may penetrate a lung. The result is a disruption of the activity of the heart and lungs and agonizing pain, to say the least, (Figure 18).

Fifth and Sixth Thoracic vertebrae: This striking point is squarely in the center of the back, at about the level of the lower ends of the shoulder blades. The spinal cord, and indirectly, the thoracic organs are under attack. This area is frequently attacked by a blow from a rifle butt used to stun or kill a sentry, (Figures 16 and 19).

Side of chest: The target area is the side of the rib cage just below the armpit, at about the same level as the fourth intercostal space. There is no particularly weak structure here, but a very powerful attack will break and dislocate the ribs, possibly driving them into the lungs. Karate blows directed to this point are almost exclusively kicks, which can be slipped in when the opponent raises his arm to ward off a high-level hand technique, (Figures 15 and 20).

43

Figure 18

Figure 18 is a diagrammatic cross section of the spine at the level of the third rib. The striking point is shown by the black arrow. Struck forcefully from behind, the rib tears away from the vertebra (white arrow) and into the chest cavity. In the course of this, the rib head severs a spinal nerve, and damages the sympathetic nerve trunk.

   a.   Thoracic vertebra
   b.   Spinal cord
   c.   Spinal ganglion
   d.   Sympathetic nerve truck (a cord of nerve tissue which runs down the length of the backbone, seen here in cross section.)
   e.   Rib

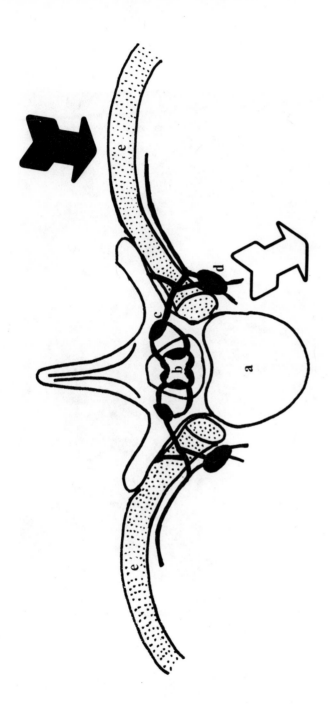

FIGURE 18

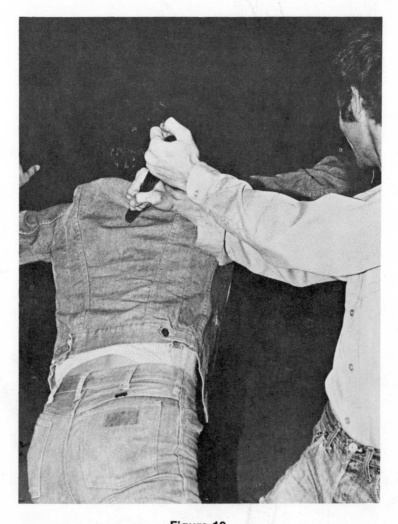

Figure 19
A potentially lethal blow to the spine (5th and 6th thoracic vertebrae) administered with the butt of a nightstick.

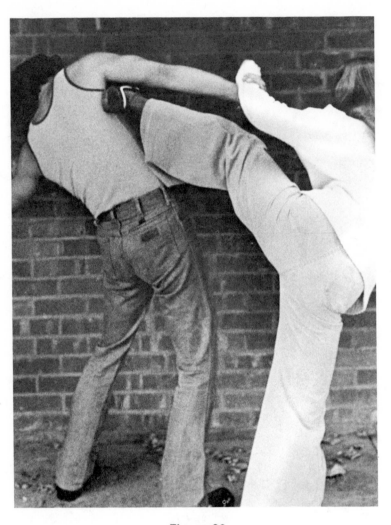

Figure 20
The kick to the side of the chest can be slipped in under a raised arm, jarring the thoracic organs and bruising several important nerves in the armpit.

Vital Points of the Lower Trunk

Celiac (solar) plexus: The soft spot just below the stomach. A relatively light blow to this area will shock the diaphragm, momentarily paralyzing it, which makes breathing difficult. Pain and giddiness result, especially in an individual who has been exercising heavily and therefore is breathing hard. A powerful blow directed straight in (rather than upward as in the case of the xiphoid process) can injure portions of the liver and stomach, producing internal bleeding, shock to some of the thoracic ganglia and unconsciousness. This striking area is not protected by either bone or muscle which makes it singularly vulnerable even to finger pokes. The end of a nightstick can produce a very dramatic effect here, (Figure 21).

Seventh intercostal space (liver): About four inches to the right of the solar plexus. The target area is the combined costal cartilages of the seventh, eighth, nineth and tenth ribs above the liver. Trauma to the liver can cause internal bleeding and possible fatal long-term metabolic dysfunction. A blow at this point will also paralyze the diaphragm temporarily, (Figure 15).

Seventh intercostal space (stomach): About four inches to the left of the solar plexus. As in the case of the previous striking point, the target is the combined costal cartilages of the lower ribs, but on the left side they overlie the stomach and spleen. The stomach may be forced to regurgitate its contents by a blow to this region. The spleen is one of the blood reservoirs of the body and can be injured relatively easily, producing internal bleeding. And, again, the diaphragm can be adversely affected by a blow to this area, (Figure 15). It is possible to force the fingers up behind the costal cartilages at this point, grasp them, and yank them outward. The sensation is indescribably unpleasant.

Eleventh intercostal space (floating ribs): The eleventh and twelfth ribs are the "floating ribs," so-called because they are not connected to the sternum by costal cartilages. They lie very low on the side of the abdomen, about four inches above the hip bones. These ribs can be broken by a relatively light blow damaging either the stomach or the liver as in the case

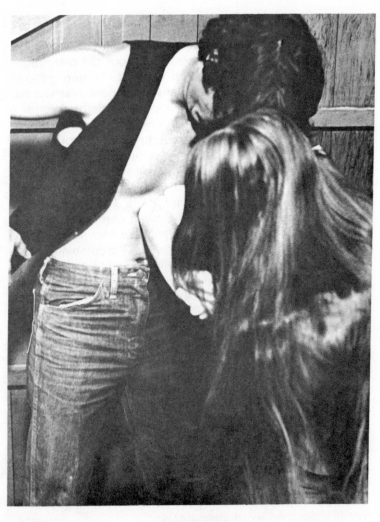

Figure 21
An elbow blow to the celiac (solar) plexus can knock the wind out of even the strongest attacker.

of the previous two striking points. Such a blow is commonly delivered from the side, traveling in toward the center of the body. This is a favorite nightstick target, (Figure 22).

Abdominal aorta and Vena cava: A knife wound anywhere in the abdomen can cause enough shock to put a man down, but this depends on the man and his state of mind. A deep thrust followed by jerking the blade sideways can sever the aorta or vena cava which lie along the backbone, resulting in massive internal bleeding and instant death, (Figure 10).

Lower abdomen: This vital point is just below the navel. A punch directed downward into the bowl of the pelvis will injure the bladder, the lower large intestine, the genitals, the femoral arteries and a profusion of spinal nerves. The pain and shock caused by a blow to this complex area is stunning.

Iliac crest: A thrust kick which lands squarely on the hip bone will badly jar an opponent, possibly injuring the nerves of the lower back. Breaking this bone, as with a heavy club, immediately puts the opponent on the ground.

Kidneys: The striking point is just to the left or right of the eleventh thoracic vertebra, partially covered by the last rib. The kidneys are very delicate organs richly supplied with blood. Their proximity to the abdominal aorta makes them particularly prone to massive hemorrhage when injured. Damage to the kidneys can cause shock and even death. This is a primary knife target since the kidneys and the renal arteries are very close to the surface and can be reached by a shallow thrust, (Figure 23).

First lumbar vertebra: There are several combat karate techniques which involve lifting an opponent up into the air and then dropping him across your bent knee, snapping his backbone at the level of the first lumbar vertebra, (Figure 16 and 24).

Fifth lumbar vertebra: This is the last vertebra above the pelvis. It articulates with the sacrum, which is essentially fused to the pelvis, so all coordinated movement between the upper and lower halves of the body pivots upon this joint. Any damage to the spine at this point will serve to weaken an opponent even if no serious damage to the spinal nerves should result, (Figure 16).

Testicles: The genitals are very delicate and are so loaded with sensory nerves that even a glancing blow to the groin can be completely debilitating. A full power blow to the scrotum

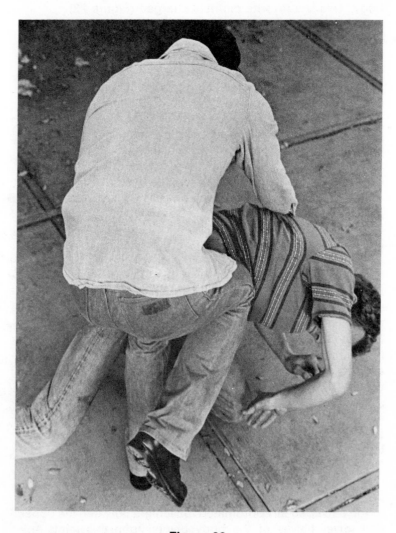

Figure 22
A knee-kick to the floating ribs is a persuasive method of keeping a grounded opponent down.

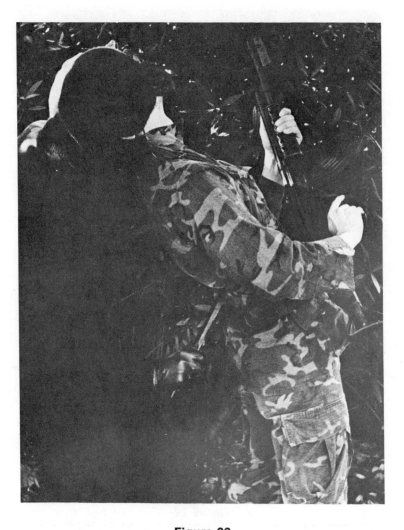

Figure 23
The stab to the kidney is the classic example of an effective, skillfully-executed knife attack.

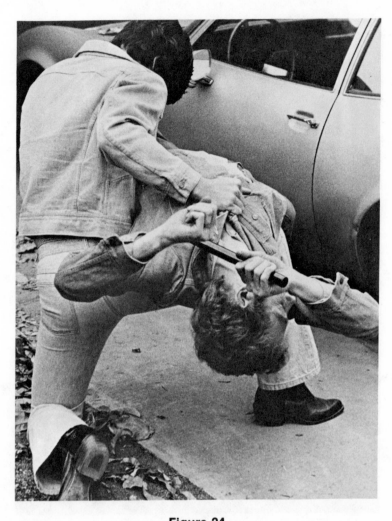

Figure 24
One of the more brutal unarmed defense techniques consists of breaking a man's back over your bent knee. The victim has been forcefully dropped across the knee from shoulder height.

54

and testes will crush these organs against the pubic bones and can result in actual castration. The drawback in using this target is that street fighters universally expect the attack and learn to defend against it. Fathers who advise their daughters to "knee the bastard in the crotch" usually haven't taken this into consideration.

The reader should be cautioned that there is a slight delay between this injury and the resulting agony. Some combat karate schools train their students to make use of the second or so between injury and collapse to catch the attacker off-guard and kill him before becoming helpless. A full second to work with is more than enough time for a desperate karateist to land several potentially lethal blows.

Coccyx: This is the tailbone, located at the tip of the spinal column beneath the sacrum. The coccyx overlies the sacral plexus where nearly all of the major nerve trunks of the hips and legs originate. In addition, the coccyx is a vestigial part of the spine and as such is innervated directly by a spinal nerve which descends from the extreme tip of the spinal cord. Fracture of the coccyx affects all the above mentioned nerves, producing agonizing pain. Fracture of the coccyx requires corrective surgery but does not endanger the life or health of the injured party.

Healing, even after surgery, is delayed and painful because the anal muscles attach to the coccyx, and pull against the fracture whenever the victim has a bowel movement, (Figures 16, 25 and 36).

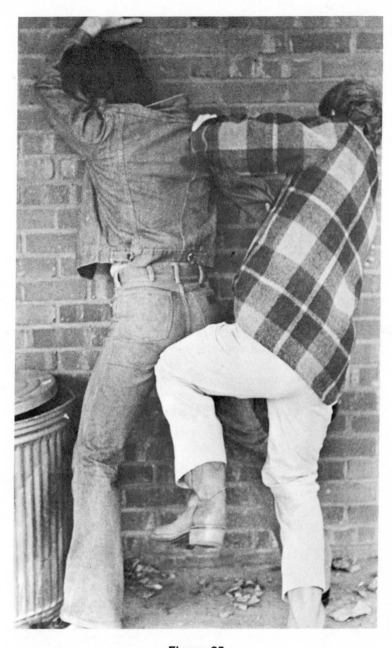

Figure 25
A knee kick to the coccyx is extremely painful and the injury takes a long time to heal.

Vital Points of the Hand and Arm

Shoulder joint: Under the proper circumstances the humerus can be twisted and torn entirely out of its socket in the shoulder. The dislocation takes the fight out of an opponent immediately.

Subaxillary bundle: There is a target located high on the inner side of the arm, about an inch down from the fold of the armpit. The brachial artery can be felt at this point, and within a fraction of an inch of this artery lie portions of several major nerves, including the radial, ulnar, and medial nerves. A sharp blow or pinch at this point will damage these nerves and temporarily paralyze the arm. A slashing cut with a knife will sever the artery and the nerves, causing permanent paralysis at the least, and death within minutes if the bleeding is not stopped, (Figure 26).

Radial nerve (lateral aspect): About halfway down the outer side of the upper arm the radial nerve is exposed where it crosses the humerus on its way from the shoulder down into the forearm. The striking point is immediately beneath the insertion of the deltoid muscle. Bruising the nerve at this point produces much the same effect as that of striking the "funny bone," i.e., a general weakening of the arm and a peculiarly debilitating pain in the arm and shoulder, (Figure 27).

Triceps muscle: The muscle on the back of the upper arm which causes the straightening of the arm at the elbow. A sharp blow, such as a knuckle blow, to the belly of the muscle will cause temporary paralysis of the arm making it very difficult for the opponent to use hand techniques effectively.

The mechanism for this is rather complex. Most of the muscles of the body operate in opposing pairs and pull against each other at all times. By stimulating one muscle and inhibiting the opposite muscle the body achieves movement. But most muscles are actually strong enough to tear their own tissue if they attempt to contract at full power when no movement is possible, such as in the case of a man trying to lift a very heavy object. To prevent injuries of this sort the body has nerves within the muscles and their tendons which sense this

Figure 26

Front of the arm.
a. Subaxillary bundle (arteries, nerve and tendons)
b. Insertion of the biceps muscle (cubital fossa)
c. Superficial branch of the radial nerve (in the mound of the forearm)
d. Inside of wrist (radial artery, flexor tendons, and medial nerve)

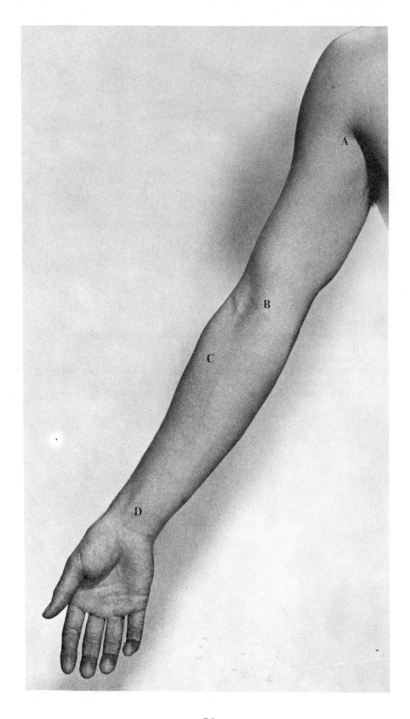

Figure 27

The back of the arm.
a. Radial nerve (just below the insertion of the deltoid muscle)
b. Triceps muscle
c. Ulnar nerve ("funny bone")
d. Superficial branch of the radial nerve (in the mound of the forearm)
e. Ulna (about one and one-half inches above the wrist)
f. Nerve pressure points of the hand

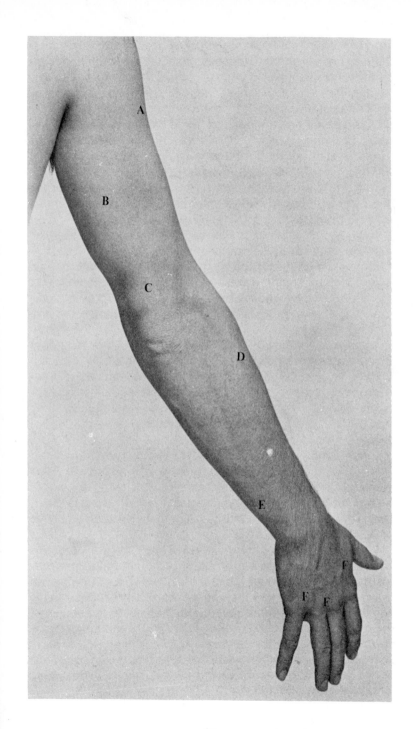

61

sort of self-inflicted damage and react by paralyzing both the injured muscle and the opposing muscle. This inhibition of the strained tissue makes it impossible for the muscle to contract strongly enough to do itself any further damage. The karate-ist can take advantage of this protective reaction by striking at the bellies and tendons of large muscles. This triggers the paralyzing reflex which then weakens not only the muscle which was attacked, but *other muscles as well.*

The triceps muscle and the radial nerve are also very vulnerable to a knife slash, as when one fighter lunges for the kill but his opponent sidesteps and slashes at the extended arm, (Figure 27).

Biceps: The belly of the bicep muscle can be bruised, or slashed with a knife, temporarily paralyzing the arm.

Cubital fossa (insertion of the biceps): The thick bundle of tendons extending down from the bicep into the hollow of the elbow can be injured by a chop, or severed by a heavy "sabre cut" with a Bowie knife. Both attacks render the arm useless, (Figure 26).

Ulnar nerve: There is a soft spot in the back of the upper arm about an inch up from the point of the elbow, beneath which lies a portion of the ulnar nerve. This is the point commonly called the "funny bone." A sharp blow at this point produces a paralyzing kind of pain in the arm and shoulder. Many armlocks depend on pressure applied to this point, (Figure 27).

Elbow joint: The striking point is the back of the straightened arm at the elbow. A relatively light blow to this spot will dislocate the elbow, breaking the arm.

Olecranon: Point of elbow. When the elbow is bent, a sharp blow on its point from a nightstick can shatter the end of the ulna, (Figure 28).

Superficial branch of radial nerve: This is the branch of the radial nerve which passes through the mound of the forearm, the muscular bulge in the top of the forearm about three inches down from the elbow. A blow to this nerve will produce a dull aching pain in the forearm and hand that results in a weakening of the muscles which control the fingers and hand. Once struck in the mound of the forearm an opponent will experience difficulty in forming a fist or grasping a weapon. This nerve center is commonly a target for a knife-hand block (chop), (Figures 26 and 27).

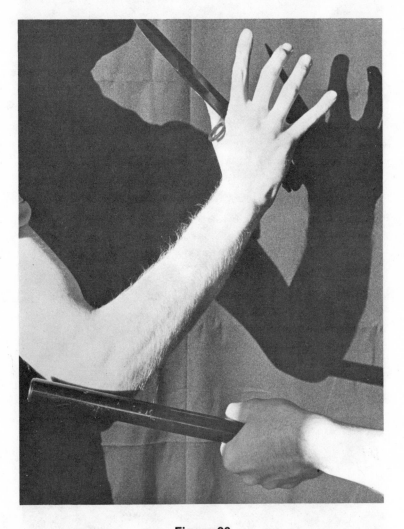

Figure 28
A nightstick blow on the tip of the elbow can chip or break the end of the
ulna, immobilizing the arm.

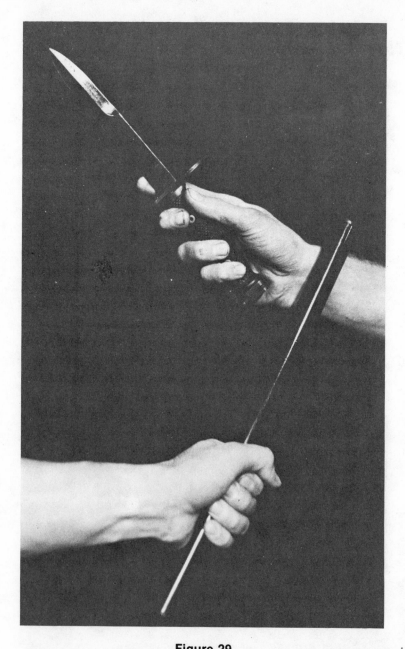

Figure 29
A club blow or karate chop to the inside of the wrist can shock the median nerve, making it difficult for the opponent to control his hand. A sharp blow here can force the hand to open involuntarily, releasing the weapon.

Median nerve: The inside of the wrist about an inch and a half up the arm from the heel of the hand. The striking point is the soft area between the radius and ulna. A blow at this point produces damage to the underlying median nerve. Digging lightly into this area with a knuckle produces an unusually intense and sickening kind of pain in the forearm, (Figures 26 and 29).

Radial artery and **Flexor tendons:** A knife slash across the inside of the wrist will sever the radial artery and several of the tendons which pull the fingers into a fist. The opponent loses the ability to grasp anything with his hand, and will pass out within thirty seconds, (according to Fairbairn) if he does not use his other hand to stop the bleeding. Therefore, a slashed wrist will effectively "disarm" an opponent. It takes about two minutes to bleed to death from this injury, (Figures 26 and 30).

Back of the wrist: About two inches up the back of the arm from the wrist joint. The median nerve can be shocked by a sharp blow at the back of the wrist, such as a knifehand chop.

Ulna: A sharp blow to the ulna, about one and one-half inches above the wrist, such as with a nightstick, will snap it in two and immobilize the arm. (The author speaks from painful experience), (Figures 27 and 31).

Wrist joint: When bent in certain ways, the wrist will lock painfully and can be broken or used as a controlling pain. Aikido students in particular are fond of wrist locks, (Figure 32).

Back of the hand: There are three vulnerable areas. The radial nerve and the ulnar nerve form a loop of nerve tissue which runs out the thumb side of the hand, across the back of the hand just behind the knuckles, and back down the little finger side of the hand. These nerves are particularly vulnerable at three points: (1) between the thumb and the index finger where the radial nerve is exposed against the side of the second metacarpal bone, (2) between the knuckles of the middle and ring fingers where the two nerves meet, and (3) along the little finger side of the fourth metacarpal where the ulnar nerve is exposed. A sharp digging blow with a yawara stick or gouging with the fingernails at these points will produce surprisingly severe pain in the hand and arm. These nerve points are usually used to break the opponent's grip on a knife or other object, (Figures 27 and 33).

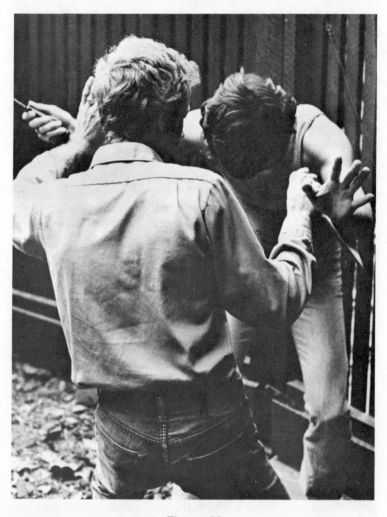

Figure 30
In this photo one fighter has tried to grab the other but has been blocked by a slash to the inside of the wrist.

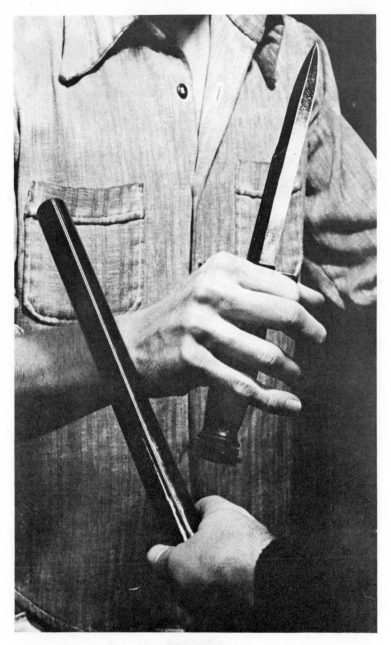

Figure 31
Baton attack to the ulna. The smaller of the two long bones of the forearm is easy to break just behind the wrist.

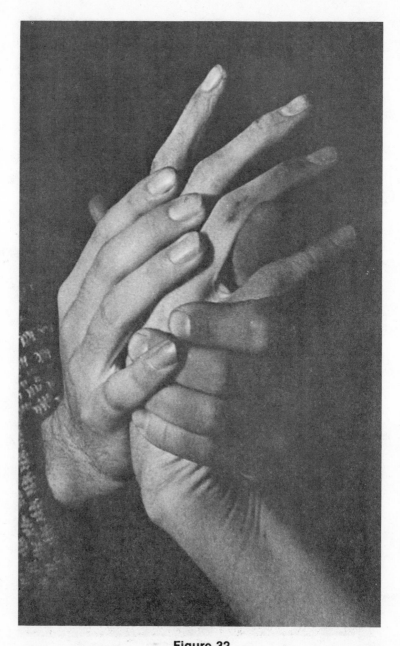

Figure 32
The wrist joint can be locked painfully and used to control an opponent with the threat of dislocation. When the wrist is forced into this position the opponent's hand involuntarily opens and drops any weapon he may be holding.

Fingers: The fingers can be "jammed" or sprained very easily, a frequently used tactic being to strike the opponent's hands to hurt his fingers and make it difficult for him to make fists. Many releases depend on spraining or breaking one or more of the opponent's fingers, (Figure 34). In knife and bayonet fighting the fingers are primary targets, and a heavy blade can actually sever them. Once the hands have been mulilated in this manner the enemy is defenseless.

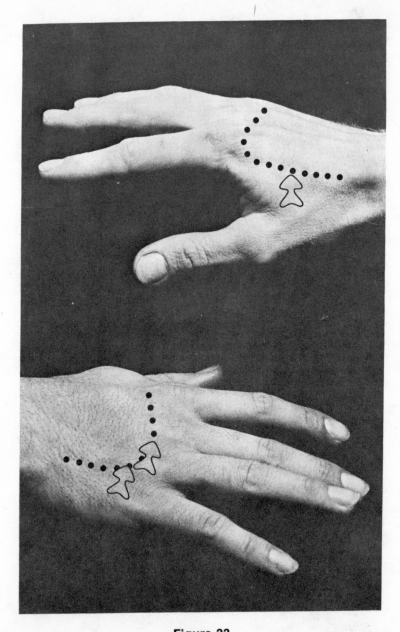

Figure 33
The nerve pressure points of the back of the hand. The dotted lines show the paths of the nerves, and the arrows indicate the three locations where the nerves can be squeezed against underlying bones by gouging with the finger-nails.

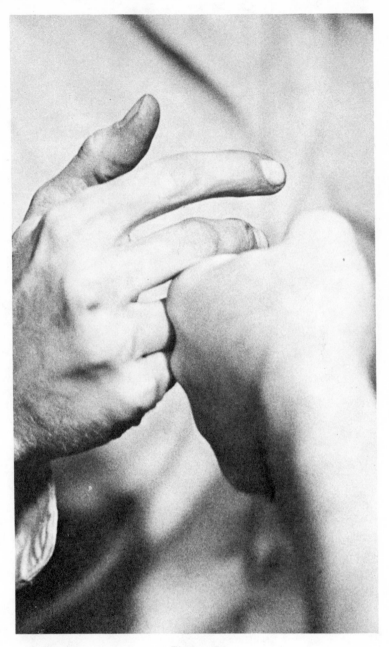

Figure 34
In a fist fight a fast punch to the opponent's relaxed fingers can sprain, break or dislocate them making the hand useless.

Vital Points of the Leg and Foot

Inguinal region: The inside front of the upper thigh, at the fold where the thigh joins the trunk. The striking point includes the first few inches of the path of the femoral nerve, the femoral artery and vein, and the genitofemoral nerve at the point where they exit the abdomen and enter the thigh. Of primary importance is the femoral nerve, which innervates the sartorius and quadriceps femoris muscles. Trauma to this nerve will paralyze or greatly weaken the thigh muscles, preventing the use of any coordinated foot techniques by the opponent. In addition, the pain generated by a blow to the femoral nerve can be sufficient to take the fight out of an opponent even if loss of muscle control does not occur. A deep gouging of the opponent's inguinal areas with your thumbs is a quick release from a bear hug even when both your arms are pinned to your sides.

A knife or bayonet injury to this area is extremely serious because of the large size and exposure of the femoral artery. Unconsciousness and death follow in seconds. Note that some military manuals have mistakenly shown this point as being almost halfway down the thigh. The true target is no lower than the level of the testicles, (Figure 35).

Sciatic nerve: The striking point is the center of the back of the thigh just below the fold of the buttocks. The largest nerve of the body, the sciatic nerve, is vulnerable at this point. The sciatic nerve gives rise to the peroneal nerve and the tibial nerve, hence a kick to the gluteal fold will interfere with muscular control of the back of the thigh and the entire lower leg and foot. The blow also produces relocated pain in the abdomen as well as pain and cramping at the point of impact, (Figures 36 and 37).

Femur: There are karate techniques, mainly kicks, which purport to snap the thighbone in two, but this takes tremendous power, (Figure 37).

Vastus lateralis: The large muscle running down the outside of the thigh. This is one part of the *quadricips femoris,* the alliance of four large muscles which extend the leg by straightening the knee. This and the next striking point . . .

Figure 35

The front view of the leg.
a. Inguinal region (femoral vein, artery and nerve)
b. Vastus lateralis
c. Rectus femoris
d. Patella (kneecap)
e. Knee joint (strike anywhere on the front and sides)
f. Deep peroneal nerve (shin)
g. Arch of the foot (right against the shin)
h. Lateral plantar nerve

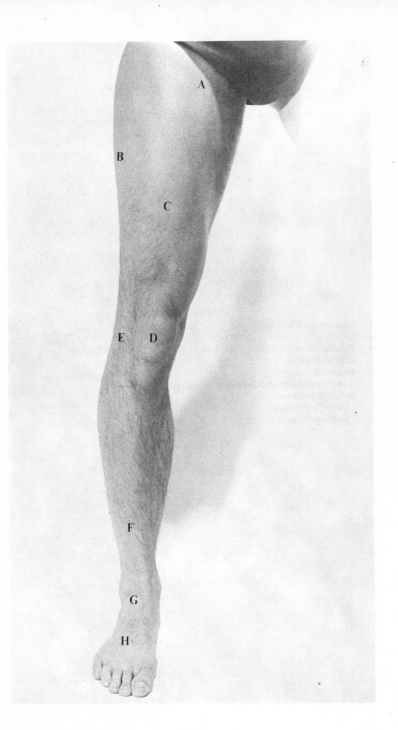

Figure 36

The rear view of the leg.
a. Coccyx
b. Sciatic nerve (within or just below the fold of the buttocks)
c. Hamstrings
d. Popliteal fossa
e. Gastrocnemius and Soleus muscles
f. Achilles tendon
g. Lateral malleolus
h. Tibial nerve and artery

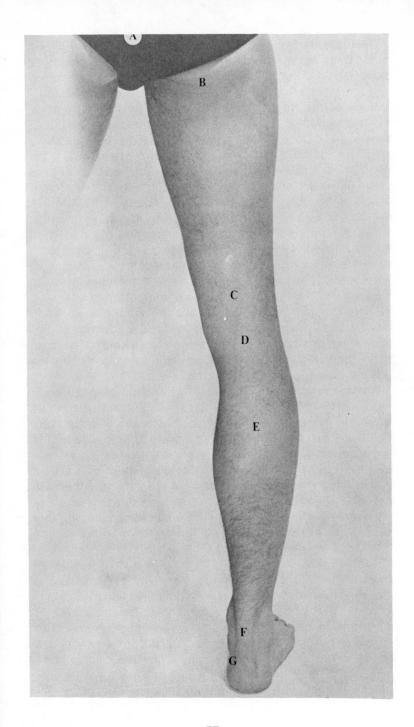

Rectus femoris: ... are both areas where a kick or club blow to the belly of the muscle will cause temporary paralysis and cramping, making it difficult for the opponent to maneuver and impossible for him to use foot techniques, (Figure 35).

Back of the thigh (the hamstrings): The biceps femoris, the semitendinosus, and the semimembranosus are three specialized muscles of the back of the thigh which collectively are known as the hamstrings. Although they are located in the thigh, these three muscles actually are attached to the bones of the pelvis and the lower leg, and do not attach to the femur at all. For this reason the hamstrings are able to both straighten the hip and also bend the knee. These are the muscles which athletes spend so much time trying to lengthen, because when the hip if fully flexed, as when attempting a high kick, the hamstrings are normally too short to allow full straightening of the knee at the same time. A blow to the bellies of these muscles will partially paralyze them, temporarily weakening the leg. Beneath these muscles lies the sciatic nerve which may also be affected by a blow to this area. Under rare conditions, the hamstrings may be presented as a knife or bayonet target. Severing them produces immediate collapse of the leg and permanent crippling, (Figures 36 and 37).

Patella or **Kneecap:** The patella is a small piece of bone which carries a tendon across the knee joint from the rectus femoris to the tibia. When the leg is extended fully and relaxed, the patella can be grasped and manipulated from side to side and up and down over the surface of the knee joint. This looseness makes the patella vulnerable to dislocation by a skillful kick which catches the lower edge of the bone at either side and drives it upward at a forty-five degree angle across the face of the knee joint. Once dislocated, the patella requires surgery before it can be relocated, and permanent injury to the mobility of the leg may result, (Figures 35 and 38).

Front or side of the knee: The knee is a very weak joint since it is held together by a number of small ligaments and little else. In addition, the knee joint connects two of the longest bones in the body, the femur and the tibia, which makes it vulnerable to blows falling anywhere in the central third of the leg. When the knee is bent it can be *broken* by a kick against either side of the joint, and when the knee is completely straight in toward the patella. The knee is particularly vulnerable because in most fighting stances this is the part of

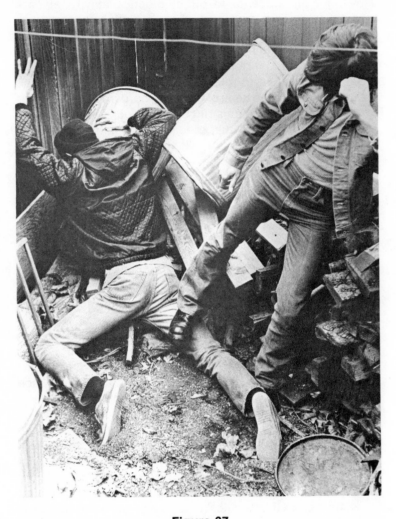

Figure 37

The photo shows an attack on the sciatic nerve and hamstring muscles intended to insure that a temporarily downed opponent stays down. In this position such a kick might easily break the femur as well.

the body closest to the opponent.

Broken knees have a reputation of not healing very well at all, and for this reason most karate instructors refrain from allowing their students to direct practice attacks at each other's knees. This is a target where a slight error can cause severe injury and permanent disability. Needless to say, in an emergency a kick to the knee will immobilize an opponent, effectively putting him out of the fight, (Figure 35).

Back of the knee (popliteal fossa): The popliteal fossa is the indentation at the back of the knee, bordered on either side by the tendons of the hamstrings. A light kick to this point will almost invariably bend the knee, abruptly bringing the opponent to a kneeling position. The tibial nerve is vulnerable at this point as well, (Figure 36).

Deep peroneal nerve: This nerve lies exposed on the surface of the tibia from a point about seven inches below the knee all the way down to the front of the ankle. Also known as the anterior tibial nerve, this nerve is vulnerable to any kicking or raking action against the front of the tibia. An unusually sharp pain results, which in addition to weakening the whole leg, also paralyzes the muscles which flex the foot and toes upward. This makes it impossible for the opponent to perform tricks involving the ball, front, or side of the foot. Severe trauma to this nerve will produce "footdrop," a condition where the toes drag on the ground with every forward step, greatly reducing the opponent's mobility, (Figure 35).

Gastrocnemius and Soleus muscles: These are the muscles of the back of the lower leg which extend the foot and which support the weight of the body when one stands on one's toes. It is interesting to note that the gastrocnemius is another of the unusual leg muscles which spans two joints, in this case the knee and the ankle joints. A kick to the back of the calf will tend to weaken and paralyze these muscles, and the tibial nerve may be injured as well, (Figure 36).

Achilles' tendon (tendo calcaneous): Any kind of stomping or raking kick to the Achilles' tendon is tantamount to a blow to the gastrocnemius and soleus muscles, since it is through this tendon that these muscles act upon the foot. Stretching of the tendon stimulates injury-sensing nerves which misinterpret the situation and inhibit the calf muscles. An attack upon the opponent's Achilles' tendon will produce pain and weakness in the opponent's legs. A knife slash here will sever the

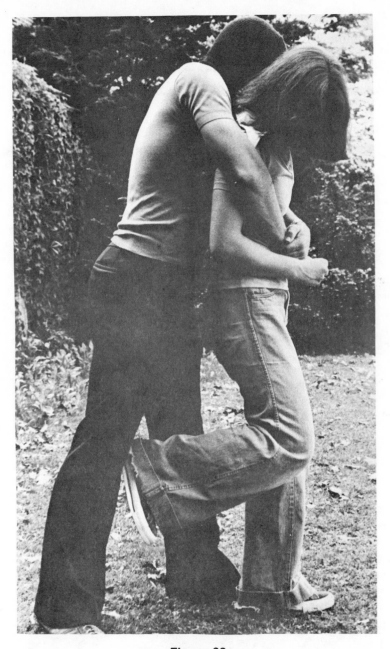

Figure 38
When embraced from behind it is very easy to attack the opponent's knees, shins and feet. Here a difficult dislocation of the kneecap is being attempted.

tendon and bring the opponent — permanently — to his knees, (Figure 36).

Lateral malleolus: This target area is the hard bony lump on the outside of the ankle, and the side of the fibula for a few inches up the leg from the ankle. The superficial peroneal nerve runs through the skin over the bone in this area, and a raking blow down the fibula will damage it. This will inhibit the muscles which control the ankle. This makes it very difficult to maintain one-point balance on the injured foot, (Figure 36).

Tibial nerve and posterior tibial artery: Immediately below the medial malleolus, which is the hard bony lump on the inside of the ankle, the tibial artery and nerve are exposed to attack where they cross the side of the first tarsal bone (the talus) on their way down into the sole of the foot. Trauma to this area produces pain in the entire leg and hip and paralyzes the posterior calf muscles, making it impossible to flex the foot downward. This is turn makes it very difficult for the opponent to support his weight on the injured foot, (Figure 36).

Arch of the foot: The target point is the instep of the foot at the base of the first and second metatarsals, where the shin meets the foot. Trauma to the arch of the foot at this point will also injure portions of the medial plantar nerve, the deep peroneal nerve and the superficial peroneal nerve. The net result is loss of coordination in the entire leg plus secondary pain in the leg and abdomen, (Figure 35).

Lateral plantar nerve: The striking point is about two inches from the point described above, at the level of the fourth and fifth metatarsals. Dislocation or fracture of these bones results in trauma to the lateral plantar nerve, another of the branches of the posterior tibial nerves, producing severe pain and partial paralysis of the lower leg, (Figure 35).

Toes: The toes, like the fingers, are easily sprained by nearly any blow which brushes across the end of the foot, such as any of a variety of blocks which might be used to nullify an opponent's kick. An untrained individual could be sufficiently distracted by this injury that he might glance downward momentarily or in some other way lose his concentration and make himself vulnerable to a more serious attack.

Vital Points of Pistol Shooting

Why should a manual of vital points include a section on pistol shooting? There is a very good reason illustrated by the following story.

In their classic combat text, *Shooting to Live,* W. E. Fairbairn and E. A. Sykes related the tale of a sergeant of police who interrupted a Chinese robber as he was holding up a rice shop in Shanghai.

> The Chinese immediately opened fire on the sergeant with an automatic pistol at about six yards, firing several shots until his pistol jammed. Fortunately, none of the shots took effect, and meanwhile the sergeant returned the fire swiftly and effectively with a .45 Colt automatic, commencing at about ten feet and firing his sixth and last shot at three feet as he rapidly closed in on his opponent. Later, it was found that of those six shots, four had struck fleshy parts of the body, passing clean through, while one bullet remained in the shoulder and another had lodged near the heart. Yet, in spite of all this, the robber was still on his feet and was knocked unconscious by the butt of the sergeant's pistol as he was attempting to escape by climbing over the counter.

The point of the story is that it is quite possible to shoot an attacker full of holes with a pistol and yet not stop him! Although there are many confounding factors to take into account, it turns out that the "stopping power" of a pistol bullet depends mainly on what part of the body is hit. In other words, there are a certain number of vital areas of the body which when hit by a pistol bullet will produce instant incapacitation. If these areas are missed though, there is no guarantee that any bullet wounds inflicted will slow the man down at all. Contrary to popular opinion, variations in bullet diameter, weight, speed and energy have much less effect on the stopping power of pistol bullets than the placement of the shot.

The previous statement calls for some justification. According to the Army Medical Department's *Wound Ballistics,* bullets of roughly the size used in modern small arms require a minimum velocity of 120 feet per second in order to penetrate human skin. Another 200 feet per second of speed is used up in penetrating a layer of bone, such as a rib, the breastbone or the braincase. Allowing a little more to account for damage to internal structures after penetration we can make the generalization that just about any kind of small arms bullet traveling faster than 400 feet per second represents a potentially lethal projectile. That pistol bullets in general are potentially lethal with standard velocities in excess of 700 feet per second is not in question. Even the lowly BB-cap traveling at 400 f.p.s. has been known to kill.

For most pistol calibers the maximum velocity of the bullet does not exceed 1200 f.p.s. At speeds between 400 and 1200 f.p.s. the bullet has a tendency to bore a hole through the body, creating a wound channel that is about the same diameter as the bullet. Damage is confined to this channel. At velocities higher than 1200 f.p.s. the bullet carries enough energy that under special circumstances much more severe wounds can result, but generally the bullet simply passes through the body. It is only after the bullet has been accelerated above 2400 f.p.s. that the high-velocity "explosive" wound becomes typical, in which a wide zone of tissue around the wound track is pulped by the passage of the bullet. No defensive handgun approaches this level.

The most complete and comprehensive investigation of the effect of various pistol calibers and bullet designs on the human body was conducted by John T. Thompson and Louis A. LaGarde over seventy years ago on behalf of the War Department. (Note that pistol and bullet designs have changed very little since then). It was their ghoulish task to fire handguns at human cadavers under controlled circumstances in search of a pistol load that would prove more effective in combat than the .38 caliber sidearm the Army was using at that time. There was some thought that when an enemy soldier is swinging a machete at your head it would be nice if your pistol would kill him instantly rather than just puncture him.

Thompson and LaGarde tested a variety of pistols and bullet designs on the cadavers and carefully evaluated the wounds produced. Their conclusions, confined to a discussion of handguns, contradicted some of the more *macho* inclinications of shooters then and today.

According to Thompson and LaGarde, the vital points of

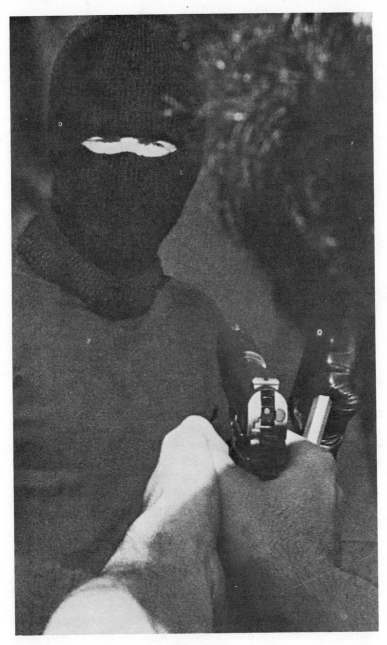

Figure 39
In combat pistol shooting, the brain is the primary target for maximum stopping power.

pistol combat shooting consists of the brain, spinal cord, and the long bones of the legs, (Figure 40). No other part of the body can be wounded by a pistol bullet in such a way as to guarantee that the victim will collapse immediately. Shots through the heart or major blood vessels can very quickly prove fatal, but collapse may not come quickly enough to prevent injury or death to the shooter.

Pistol wounds through the lungs, although commonly regarded as fatal, cannot be depended upon to drop a man in his tracks. This is true also of wounds in other fleshy parts of the body. To test for "shock" effects due to multiple wounds, which the cadavers didn't show very well, Thompson and LaGarde fired rapid bursts of shots into the chests of living cattle. The idea was to determine what effect multiple shots through the lungs had on "stopping power" as measured by the number of shots it took to make a steer collapse. They found that ten .30 caliber Luger bullets (93 gr., 1420 f.p.s.) through the lungs did not upset the steers at all. The animals turned their heads to see what had caused all the noise, but showed no sign of distress. (This says something about the effectiveness of small caliber sidearms and also about how stupid a steer is). .45 caliber and larger bullets should drop the steers, but it usually took four or five shots.

As for "knock down," there is probably no greater area of misinformation in the whole subject of stopping power. According to Newton's third law, the detonation of the powder charge in a pistol must push the pistol backward as forcefully as it pushes the bullet forward. Therefore, if the recoil transmitted to the shooter's body from the gun is not enough to knock him off his feet, then it follows that the energy absorbed by the victim's body when struck by the bullet will not be enough for a "knock down" either. In his *Textbook of Pistols and Revolvers*, Julian S. Hatcher demonstrated this point with a series of calculations showing that a standard military .45 ACP bullet carries only enough energy to knock a man backward at a rate of a little less than two inches per second. This is next to nothing. Fairbairn and Sykes, authors of *Shooting to Live*, related their attempts to examine the "knock down" potential of pistol bullets by allowing themselves to be shot at while holding a bullet-proof shield. They reported that in all cases the force transmitted to them through the shield was negligible. The ability of modern kevlar body

86

armor to stop .44 magnum bullets at point-blank range without knocking the wearer off his feet is further proof of this point, if any is needed.

Thompson and LaGarde concluded that any pistol load in general use could penetrate the brain case and produce an instantly lethal wound of the brain. It was also found that although some of the higher velocity bullets (comparable to today's magnums) could produce explosive brain wounds there was no need for the added destruction. A .22 bullet in the brain will stop a man just as quickly as blowing his skull apart. Much the same conclusion was applied to the case of explosive wounds of the long bones of the legs, caused by high-velocity pistol bullets. Less energetic bullets were capable of fracturing these bones and producing instant incapacitation, and the explosive effect contributed little. In fact, the researchers tried actual exploding bullets, filled with black powder and a primer, but concluded that the wounds produced were not very different from those produced by high-velocity bullets, and therefore did not contribute much to stopping power.

The researchers found that larger pistol bullets in general produced more dangerous wounds since the wound channel was large in diameter and did not close easily when the various layers of skin and muscle re-arranged themselves after wounding. This promoted greater bleeding in wounds caused by large diameter bullets.

Pistol bullets of all types including soft lead, hollow point, and dum-dum completely failed to expand regardless of velocity unless they hit bone or solid cartilage. Soft lead bullets in a flat-point (wadcutter or semi-wadcutter) shape were judged fractionally more effective in producing wounds because they tended to catch on bones and cut into arteries in circumstances where jacketed or round-nosed bullets would glance off.

In general, Thompson and LaGarde concluded that the available pistol ammunition they tested did not differ much in terms of stopping power, although there were significant differences in penetration and general killing power. Wounds in the brain, spinal cord, and long bones of the legs would reliably stop a man regardless of the bullet employed, but for non-vital areas they somewhat facetiously suggested that a *three-inch diameter bullet* would be necessary for reliable stopping power.

Figure 40

This diagram illustrates the vital areas of combat pistol shooting as defined by Thompson and LaGarde. For absolute "stopping power" only the brain, spinal cord and the long bones of the legs can be wounded in such a way as to guarantee that the victim will drop immediately to the ground. The heart and associated major blood vessels present another vital target, but some individuals will be able to stay on their feet for several seconds after being wounded in these organs. For the situation in which all resistance must be extinguished immediately, the brain is both the most effective target and the largest.

The reader should bear in mind that in a gun fight when time is the critical factor the old rule of firing into the center of the body is still good advice. These vital areas are for occasions when the shooter has that extra split-second in which to take aim.

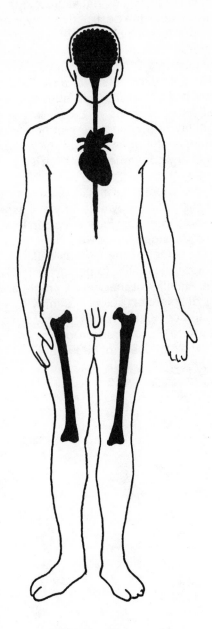

FIGURE 40

One aspect of pistol combat at close quarters that may have been overlooked is the destructive power of the muzzle blast, which can produce a more serious wound than the bullet itself if the pistol is fired in contact with the victim's body. That is a tricky business, admittedly, since there is always the possibility that the pistol will suffer a ruptured barrel if fired with the muzzle against flesh. Still, after contemplating some of the ghastly photographs in LaGarde's *Gunshot Injuries,* it is a possibility that cannot be lightly dismissed. One photo, for instance, is of a man who put the muzzle of a .30-'06 rifle in his mouth and committed suicide. It is a picture of a headless man.

The reader should not finish this essay without being reminded that stopping power is only one aspect of pistol bullet effectiveness. Other considerations can have as much or more importance as stopping power, depending on the circumstances. The effect of the various calibers, powders, bullets and pistols on the ability to penetrate barriers, on accuracy, and on the stability of the bullet in flight are quite important. The point of this discussion is simply to emphasize that in hand-to-hand combat in which the pistol may be employed, a bullet fired into a vital portion of the enemy's anatomy will drop him. One that does not hit a vital point *might* drop him . . . *or he might just keep coming.*

Further Reading

Almost all manuals of hand-to-hand combat, self-defense, and oriental or European martial arts contain at least a short section on vital points. Frequently these treatments are very incomplete and full of misinformation. Military manuals in particular are very poor sources of information about vital points.

For general anatomy, nothing beats the classic text:

Gray, Henry. 1973. *Anatomy of the Human Body,* 29th edition. Ed. by Charles Mayo Goss. Lea and Febiger, Philadelphia.

For a detailed treatment of potential injuries due to twenty-four formal karate attacks, see

Adams, Brian. 1969. *Medical Implications of Karate Blows.* 128 p. il., A.S. Barnes and Co., New York.

Fairbairn's knife-fighting "timetable of death" appears in

Fairbairn, W. E. 1942. *Get Tough!* ix + 121 p. il., Paladin Press, Boulder.

The authorities cited in the section on pistol stopping power include:

LaGarde, Louis A. 1914. *Gunshot Injuries.* William Wood and Co., New York.

Hatcher, Julian S. 1936. *Textbook of Pistols and Revolvers.* Small-Arms Technical Publishing Company, Marines, Onslow County, North Carolina.

Fairbairn, W. E. and E. A. Sykes. 1942. *Shooting to Live.* xiv + 96 p. il., Paladin Press, Boulder.

Medical Department, War Department. 1927. *Medical Department of the United States Army in the World War: v.ii, Surgery,* pt. 1, *General Surgery, Orthopedic Surgery, Neurosurgery,* xxiv + 1324 p. il. 7 pl. 1 tab.
L.C. card SG 27-47   W44.19:11/1

Army Medical Service, Defense Department. 1962. *Wound Ballistics.* Editor-in-chief James (John) Boyd Coates, Jr.; editor for wound ballistics, James C. Beyer. xxxix + 883 p. il. (Office of the Surgeon General).
L.C. card 62-60002   D104.11:W91

The U.S. Government publications can be found on the shelves of any official government depository.